Lifestyle Mapping

Chart Your Path for Living Healthfully

Frank A. Lucas, PhD, cNHC

Published in the United States of America

ISBN 979-8-89395-926-0 (SC)

Frank A. Lucas Publishing
222 West 6th Street
Suite 400, San Pedro, CA, 90731
https://creatingradianthealthpublishing.com/

Ordering Information and Rights Permission:

Quantity sales. Special discounts might be available on quantity purchases by corporations, associations, and others. For details, contact the publisher at the address above.

For Book Rights Adaptation and other Rights Permission. Call us at toll-free 1-888-945-8513 or send us an email at admin@stellarliterary.com.

To change the way things are, you must change the thing you do. People often miss the root cause(s) of declining or failing health.

Lifestyle Mapping helps you discover the habits and patterns that are producing physical decline, sickness, and/or disease.

The journal will help you chart your course back to radiant health.

Welcome to Lifestyle Mapping

This may be the best investment in time you'll ever spend!

You will learn:

1. Who is responsible for protecting you from sickness or declining health.
2. How you can protect or create health and well-being – naturally!

You, or someone you love, will benefit mightily from what you're about to learn.

These five lessons, your analysis using lifestyle mapping, and the adjustments you make, may change your life – forever.

Enjoy your journey into the World of Lifestyle Medicine.

Dedication

This guide is dedicated to the millions of people
Who are trapped in the endless cycle of declining and failing health.

Contents

Preface

The world is a dangerous place. Sometimes, it's an injury, or a terrible infection. Other times it is just bad luck – something "just happens" that changes a life, forever – sad but true.

On the other hand, there are millions of poor souls needlessly suffering from neglecting their bodies. There's a friend, a loved one - someone who, if they could - would change the way things are – making better choices – doing things differently.

And unfortunately, there are millions more people on the same, well-worn path: disregarding the signals that things are not right!

98.5% of Americans aren't healthy, they're just NOT SICK.

1. Obesity is replacing smoking as the #1 killer of Americans.
2. Indigestion and constipation are at epidemic levels.
3. Joint pain and stiffness plague millions of people.
4. The use of HRT is being discouraged because of cancer risks.
5. More and more infections are antibiotic resistant.
6. Health care costs are at record levels – and climbing!

Pharmacy shelves are lined with antacids, headache tablets, sinus tablets, laxatives, allergy tablets, pain relievers plus hundreds more - to deal with these inconveniences.

Your body is sending you signals that it needs help! Doing nothing will only compound the situation. You'll have a choice. The decision boils down to two choices: pay for sickness or invest in health.

Either way, the choice affects the rest of your life – just differently.

Understand, you have the most to gain by staying or becoming healthy,. . . or lose when you are not.

Managing your most valuable asset, your good health – just makes sense!

There's a warning we've all heard hundreds of times:

"Insanity is doing the same thing over and over again, and expecting a different outcome."

You decide - it's your life – it's your choice.

Introduction to: Lifestyle Mapping

What Does Goldilocks Know That You Need to Know?

Remember the Goldilocks fable about a little girl getting caught trespassing into the home of a family of three bears? Too much, too, little, just right.? Choices have consequences.

There you have it – The Goldilocks Dilemma.

It's the same dilemma facing people trying to navigate our modern world. Too much, too little, just right and choices have consequences.

- **Let's start with some realities you can't control.**

There are 24 hours in a day.

A day has 2 parts.

1. **Sunlight** (Day), which begins shortly before sunrise and ends shortly after sunset.
2. **Darkness** (Night), which begins shortly after sunset and ends shortly before sunrise.

There are two types of Animals:

1. Animals that are active during the day and sleep at night are known as **diurnal.**
2. Animals that are active during the night and sleep during the day are **nocturnal**.

Humans are diurnal – with 2 distinct metabolic functions:

1. **Daytime** - Catabolic metabolism.
   Catabolism is the destructive metabolic process that breaks down large more complex molecules to burn energy necessary for various functions of the body.
2. **Nighttime** - Anabolic metabolism.
   Anabolism is the constructive metabolic processes that support the growth of new cells, the maintenance of body tissues, and the storage of energy for future use.

Important: Doing daytime activities during nighttime inhibits anabolic functions; slowing or stopping the repair – replace - self-cleansing cycles of the human body.

- **Finding Your "In-Balance Sweet Spot".**

These two diagrams represent your Goldilocks' Dilemma: Too much, too little. Just right.

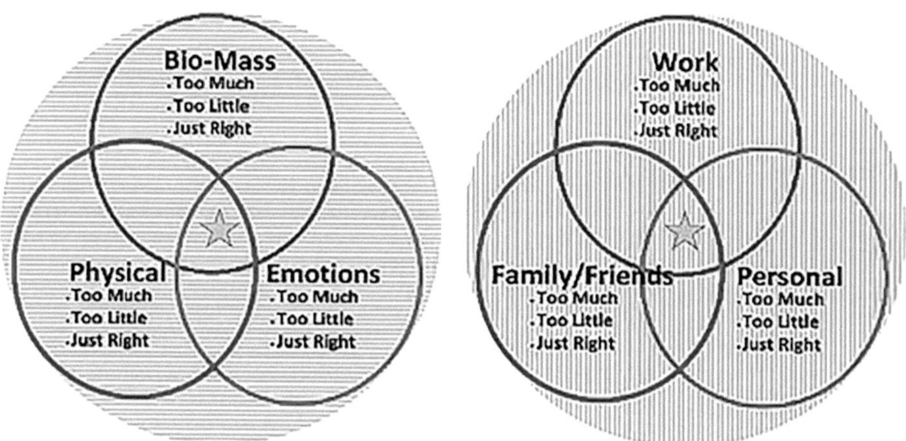

There is a tendency to separate these factors, when, in fact, they are interconnected. They, individually or together, contribute to the 4 health conditions in which people will find themselves – over time.

Choices, information overload, confusion reign our lives when balance should rule the day.

Lifestyle Mapping seeks to show you where you've lost your sweet spot.

1. There's only 24 hours in your day.
   Question. How are you spending them?
2. There's Water, Fish, Birds, Beasts and Plants on Earth for humans to eat.
   Question. Are you consistently consuming them – in balance?
3. **You're a Human Being.** You aren't the fastest, nor strongest creature in the forest.
   Question. How are you using your body?

- **Before we move forward, some definitions are in order.**

There are 4 states of health in the 21st Century.

They are: Healthy, Not Sick, Declining Health, Failing Health.

1. **Healthy**, for most people, it is the delusion that their state of "being healthy" is a forever thing. (In reality, it's a state of ignorant bliss.)
2. **Not Sick**, is a state of "soldiering on". It's getting up, every morning, even though you don't feel like it. IMPORTANT: This is the exact point where an ounce of prevention is worth a pound of cure!
3. **Declining Health** is a state of inconvenience, punctuated with the delusion that a remedy, drug store or a prescription, can make the inconvenience go away.
4. **Failing Health** is a state of disbelief, punctuated with the delusion that some medical, non-medical or spiritual intervention can make the misery and suffering go away.

The inter-connectivity between your state of health with Ven 1 and Ven 2 is unavoidable.

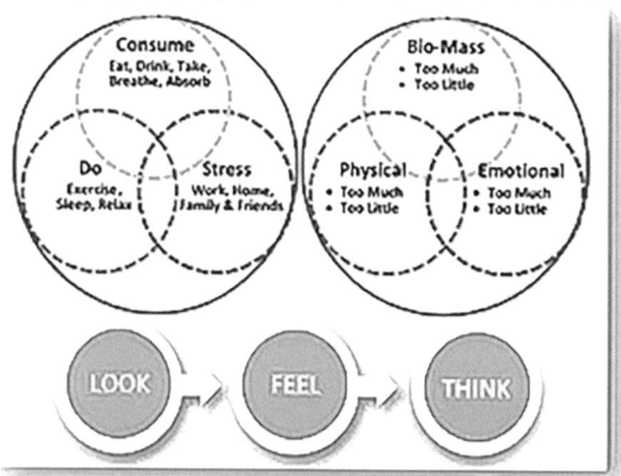

A person who finds themselves on this predictable path of declining health will experience big changes at work, in their family life and a decline in their physical and emotional well-being.

And, when the predictable happens – their state of health is in full-blown decline – people are bombarded with advice and advertisements that support the false belief that technology will erase the story that is unfolding.

Here's Another Goldilocks Moment: <u>Health Isn't Permanent</u>!

People falsely believed their health is permanent, that health happens automatically, that a fix for the problem is one phone call to their doctor away.

In a perfect world people wouldn't face this dilemma because:

- the air and water would be pristine,
- the nutritional thresholds, necessary to sustain a healthy body, would be met from the food that is consumed,
- personal and interpersonal interactions would be void of conflict, and Mary Poppins would make your decisions for you.

Oh well – the world isn't perfect. The air and water could be better, commercial food products aren't what they're trumped up to be, people aren't nice to one another – all the time, and Mary Poppins isn't on-call to make your boo-boo go away.

So, It's Up to You. You only need to know 4 rules to help you stay or become healthy:

1. Let your conscience be your guide.
2. What you do occasionally won't hurt you – it's what you do every day that helps you.
3. What you don't know can hurt you.
4. Ignorance is not bliss – nor an excuse - because your choices have consequences.

On matters of diet: Don't make perfect be the enemy of good!

- Eat as close to a balanced diet as possible, then plug the holes with fundamental nutritional supplements.
- Eat lots of differently colored above ground veggies and 2 hard fruits – every day.
- Avoid "the white stuff": white flour, sugar, starchy vegetables, salt, and tropical fruit.
- Drink Water: the calculation is: your body weight divided by 2 in ounces – every day.

On matters of supplements consider this: Your body maintains and heals itself using the "stuff" it gets from the food you eat and the water your drink. There are fundamental nutritional supplements to help fill general gaps in your diet; however, caution is the watch word.

Know this: Supplements fill gaps in your diet, so use them as such.

You should:

- Avoid the "hype" in the media and advertising because there are NO SILVER BULLETS.
- Be sure of your sources of information and products.
- Buy the highest quality possible because, in most cases, price is an indication of what you are getting.

Buying and using the right stuff sure beats the false hope that someone or something will be there to fix what you have broken – because everyone knows there aren't any magic bullets – don't they?

It's Your Life – It's Your Choice.

Lessons in Lifestyle Living

- **Living life is simple – it's just not easy . . .** especially when you consider all the opinions, advertising and outright misinformation that exasperate the process of living.

Here's the BIG question for you to consider:

"*Why have people relinquished the responsibility for staying and becoming healthy to strangers?*"

I was asked once during a healthcare interview:

"*What's the final message you would like to share with the listeners?*"

Since the interview was quite specific, I had to think for a minute.

After a brief pause, I said:

"*Learn to love your body. It's time for the person who has the most to gain – or lose – to take responsibility.*"

I'm not sure if the audience saw, but the interviewer's jaw dropped open just before he signed off.

That was several years ago, but the issue we discussed hasn't changed: Medical healthcare is good at what it's good at - but it's not limitless.

People need to take responsibility for the "easy stuff" and let Medicine handle what it's good at - infections, injuries, trauma, and surgery.

The purpose of Lifestyle Mapping is to introduce you to the fundamentals of "Loving your body and treating it with due respect" - because it's the only one you'll ever get.

It's not the end-all.

It's a place to start your journey on your life-long love affair with your most valuable asset – your body.

Enjoy the ride!

Lesson 1: Health Care vs Sick Care

- **Are You Healthy or Medically Healthy?**

There is a difference between true health and being treated medically for symptoms and sickness. Which one would you prefer?

1st let's start with some definitions.

Traditional Medicine is sick care.

- It's a reactive approach to declining health, sickness, and disease.
- It's finding a doctor for prescription(s), management, and treatment(s).

Natural Holistic medicine is Health Care.

- It's a proactive approach for protecting and improving health.
- It's using lifestyle, diet, and supplements to support and/or improve your well-being.
- It's creating holistic health.

Next, let's add some facts.

The top six causes of death are:

1. Heart Disease
2. Stroke
3. Cancer
4. Chronic Respiratory Disease
5. Diabetes
6. Obesity

(All preventable and, if addressed early, reversible).

Countless millions of people will endure seemingly endless years of suffering monetary and mental anguish, before they succumb to these killers.

Almost everyone who receives the bad news that they have "it", will spring into action.

Seeking out the "best medical attention money can buy".

And, when their insurance runs out, they mortgage themselves, to the hilt, so they can keep on fighting "the good fight" – clinging to whatever is left of their lives.

And, if they are lucky enough to survive the medical ordeal, must have their condition managed, for the rest of their lives, to prevent its return, which in and of itself is another costly affair.

But all this suffering and expense may be preventable – if only they would …

At this point, 99% of you will stop reading because you think it won't happen to you, so, good luck.

But, when it does, just remember, you were warned.

So, please, keep reading. There's a lot more you need to learn . . .

For the rest of you who kept reading, write this down:

Poor Nutrition = Poor Health. Good Nutrition = Good Health.

• No one lives forever, but your body can live, healthfully, until you die – and you control that.

Granted, there are accidents during birth, unavoidable injuries, and bad luck, but – always remember this – your body has the ability to work around the clock, 24/7 - to protect, energize, repair, replace every cell – until it can't.

It needs - and deserves – the tools, your love, and your respect to keep it happening.

• Packaged and processed convenience food is killing us. •

Your body does not benefit when you consume flavor enhancing chemicals, salt, sugar, and preservatives.

When you add in the generous amount of fast food that people consume every day, it is easy to understand why there is an explosion of these chronic diseases.

The U.S. Department of Agriculture and the U.S. National Cancer Institute report:

"Americans are failing to get the vegetable and fruit nutrition needed for optimal health."

They point out: *"... more than 60% of Americans fail to reach the minimum recommendation of 5 servings of differently colored vegetables/fruit per day – let alone the preferred recommendation – eating the 9 to 13 servings per day that it takes to promote optimum health."*

The Journal of the American Dietetic Association (September 2006) reports that:

> *". . . the dietary habits of certain studied groups were especially bad.*
>
> *. . . Boys 14-18: less than 1% reached the 5-a-day minimum target for vegetables & fruit. Women 51-70: the number was 17%. Other groups fared poorly too, prompting researchers to comment:*
>
> *"A large portion of the U.S. population needs to increase their vegetable and fruit intake if the minimum recommendations are to be met."*

• Don't Wait to Close the Barn Door Until After the Horse Runs Away.

The formulae are simple:

1. **Poor nutrition equals poor health** with a greater likelihood you will suffer with and die from one of these chronic diseases.
2. **Good nutrition equals good health** with a greater likelihood you can avoid these chronic diseases.

The U.S. Center for Disease Control, the U.S. Food and Drug Administration, the American Heart Association, the U.S. National Cancer Institute, and most major health authorities agree: ". . . *whole food diet is one our best weapons in the fight against chronic disease."*

Whole foods contain the powerful protector nutrients that are our best weapons in the fight against chronic disease.

- Eating a variety of vegetables and fruit helps you control your weight and your blood pressure.
- The fiber in whole grain foods can help lower your blood cholesterol and help you feel full, which may help you manage your weight.
- Vegetables, fruit, and grains contain a number of nutrients, to help reduce the risk of cancer.
- Eating non-starchy vegetables (those that grow above the ground) of different color and variety can help prevent diabetes.
- Eating fish containing omega-3 fatty acids, (salmon, trout, and herring) twice a week, may help lower your risk of death from coronary artery disease.

• **One Final Thought**

In a perfect world, our food would be our medicine. You could consume everything your body needs to grow old while enjoying the benefits of good health.

Our world isn't perfect, so do the best you can.

- Moderate your consumption of convenience and fast food.
- Eat more vegetables that grow above ground and fruit for between meal snacks.
- Drink more water (at least 8 – eight-ounce glasses) – less soda, coffee, and tea.
- Then, consider using well-crafted nutraceutical supplements to fill the gap in your diet between what you are eating and what you should be consuming to promote and maintain your health.

Write this down and look at it frequently.

To change the way things are, you must change the things you do.

And if you feel that your body is less than healthy, it is likely that one or more of the usual culprits - poor diet, stress, lack of rest and relaxation - could be stealing your health.

Consider changing your lifestyle and using a nutraceutical supplement to restore your wellbeing.

Here are 5 areas affecting your health to consider:

1. Poor Diet
2. Obesity
3. Constipation
4. Digestion
5. Parasite and Toxins

. . . for which supplements are helpful.

It is, after all, better to invest in health than it is to pay for sickness.

Lesson 2: Do Something Different

• Having Health Issues? Try Something Different!

Recently, I heard an interesting sermon. The talk was, of course, about religion, but while I was listening, it seemed to me that the message applies to lots of things.

It applies to health – specific health complaints and/or declining and failing health.

The basic message was:

- Ignorance → leads to → no discipline → leads to → vulnerability.
- Knowledge → leads to → self–discipline → leads to → protection

Putting 2 and 2 together, I decided to share these 2 nuggets about holistic health with you:

- Most people's health is declining because they are doing it to themselves. . . and they don't even know they are!
- Why? Because staying or getting healthy is simple – it's just not convenient!

I can understand how people get caught in the convenience trap, too.

If I've heard it once, I've heard it a thousand times: "*Between work, the kids, trying to keep up the house – I don't have the time!*"

Here's a typical day for many people:

Busy Lifestyle

→ **Rush** to get ready, get the kids fed and off to school – and yourself to work.

→ **Rush** back home to pick up the kids from school or the sitter, get the kids to their activities.

→ **Rush** back home to feed the family. Help the kids with homework. Attend to your homework, pay the bills, catch the news, try to get some sleep before it starts again.

Too Much Stress

→ Commuting, deadlines, interruptions, emergencies, bosses, colleagues, fast food and skipping meals.

Questionable Diet

→ You need to save time and money, so you: Buy meals and snacks that are on sale over the weekend.

Then, during the week

→ Open, heat and eat something because you think they are easier and faster than it is to try to plan, shop for and prepare a meal.

You might even look at the label to see if it says it has "healthy stuff" in it.
→ But, if you're like most people, you'll miss the back label that itemizes the salt, sugar and chemical additives that enhance the color and flavor of the manufactured product(s) that you're buying.

You know these 2 facts, but they bear repeating:

1. Your body depends on a consistent flow of nutrition and water to stay healthy.
2. Stress kills, but it takes a terrible toll on your health before it does.

Ask yourself these 3 questions:

1. What will you do, if "they" get sick?
2. What will "they" do if you can't do it anymore?
3. Or worse, you're not there at all?

You may not like it, but the answers are:

1. You'll have even more responsibilities and expenses than you have now.
2. You'll be a burden on them or, at least, they'll worry about you.
3. They will move on!

Write this down: Those bags, boxes & cans you're buying are manufactured products – are not food. Manufactured foods are true to their product advertising message: **fast, easy, filling, and cheap.**

Packaged foods are produced to attract your attention with packaging, have a long shelf life, make you want more, sell as cheaply as possible. **They do it very well.**

Nutrition Ain't Part of the Plan!

Processing the food destroys some or most of the nutrition, if there was any in it to start with. Instead, packaged and processed food replaces nutrition with chemicals to make it look and taste better.

And those fun and easy cereals, juices, and snacks that you and your kids consume are guilty, too....

- **Who's Doing What to Whom?**

Here's the truth: You're buying and consuming that stuff.

The key to staying healthy or becoming healthy is: Change your habits! Eat for health instead.

You might even be able to stop worrying about why: your kids are having trouble in school, you or your spouse is agitated, lethargic, or heavy, because all of it may be symptoms of your manufactured food diet.

And, by the way, a healthy diet is cheaper because you're not likely to be hungry and snacking all the time!

Here's where to start.

1st, do the best you can with home-cooked, fresh food meals; then fill the gap with a few basic supplements.

2nd, once you've started eating for health, add a little more specific nutrition, to make up for all those years of neglect, with nutritional supplements for specific needs.

3rd, if you are experiencing declining or failing health, don't despair, your body is fully capable of healing itself, if it has enough time and the right nutrition. Here is an example of levels of natural intervention that may help your body begin to heal itself. Just remember . . .

It's easier said than done. Staying or becoming healthy is simple, it's just not easy – that's because change is never easy!

Change is an act of contrition. In this case, it is the point when you realize that some, or most of the rules that have guided your lifestyle, work and diet are false and, in fact, they are harming your well-being.

Some people "get it" sooner than others. They make the changes it takes to stay or become healthy.

So, if this makes sense to you …

Instead of making a New Year type resolution – that we both know never works. . . start with changing one thing – then, after a while, move to the next.

For example, one of the easiest habits to change is to **stop skipping breakfast**.

- The quickest way to do that is to start eating breakfast instead of brewing coffee and toasting bread.
- If you're positive that you don't (or can't) have the time, you can start mixing a nutritious shake and drinking on the way to work. (Instead of waiting in line for a cup of Starbucks Latte Supremo.)
- **Once you see how much better you feel,** start making time in the morning to prepare a breakfast meal like The Perfect Breakfast (see recipe page 27).

Then, maybe you can change your TV snacking habit. Stop opening the bags of snacks – eat a cored apple or pear with a sprinkle of cinnamon instead. Why not try it?

• **The secret to changing your conditions of health is in your habits.**

You need simply to exchange the habits that contribute to declining or failing health with habits that sustain or improve your health – one or two at a time.

Certainly, there are methods that can help you move faster if your needs are greater. But rest assured, for life-long change, adjusting or changing your dietary habits is imperative, so start there.

Over the years, I've witnessed too much needless worry and sickness.

And I've seen and heard the toll it takes on families, too.

Let me assure you, all of this is mostly avoidable – and often reversible!

Knowledge and self-discipline are all it takes to possess the protection that will help you live a long healthy life.

Lesson 3: Balance Your Diet

The least understood health concept is: "The Balanced Diet".

It's too bad, because virtually all the recommendations emanating for the "medical experts" are predicated on the assumption that you are eating the nutrition recommended by the "Balanced Diet".

When asked, most people will tell you they eat "pretty good."

But the fact is they are not eating anywhere near the nutrition the body needs to stay healthy.

What people are consuming is a conglomeration of processed, preserved, packaged and convenience food products that, thanks to advertising, are masquerading as food.

Joel Wallach, MD, DVM dramatizes this issue, in his controversial presentation **"Dead Doctors Don't Lie"**, when he explains:" ***. . . if you're bringing home bags of cans, boxes and bags of food, from the supermarket, you would be better off throwing away the contents and eating the packaging.*"**

There is a litany of health concerns that are directly attributable to this blind spot regarding what people are consuming. The difference between what you are consuming and what your body needs, to be healthy and flourish, leads to the predictable decline in health that is plaguing adult men, women and now teens and children.

While the medical community has ascribed any number of names for the symptoms afflicting their patients, most of their complaints boil down to a single diagnosis: Hand to Mouth Disease.

The following chart may help you demystify the "Balanced Diet", the health implication, and the dietary source(s).

Approximate Nutrient Composition of the Body with Corresponding Dietary Recommendations	**Diet Related Health Challenges**
Water: 55%+ Drink ½ your body weight, in ounces, everyday	**Being Overweight**
Protein: 20% **Lean Meat** (beef, pork, chicken) 1-3 servings/week; **Fish**: 2-4 servings/week.	**Obesity** **Indigestion** **Auto-toxification**
Above Ground Vegetables; unlimited (5 servings/day minimum).	**Declining Health**
Fruit: 1-4 servings/day.	**Frequent Illness**
Beans, Peas, Lentils: 1-3 servings/day.	**Arthritis**
Fat: 15% Oils, nuts, seed: 1-9 servings/day **	**Premature Aging**
Minerals: 5% **FYI:** Plants are the source for all the minerals on which the body depends. Your diet dictates the rate at which minerals are replenished.	**Acidosis** **Menopause** **Andropause**
Carbohydrates: 2%* Recommendation: Whole Grain: 4-11 servings/day.	**Allergies**
Vitamins: less than 1% *	

* Source: Nutrition Almanac, Nutrition Search, Inc, McGraw-Hill, p.109
** Source: University of Michigan Integrative Medicine Dept.

• **Confused about serving size? This reference should help you.**

The secret to serving size is in your hand.

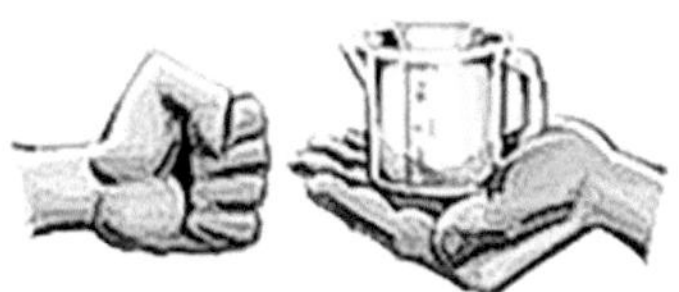

A fist or cupped hand = 1 cup

1 cup = 1½-2 servings of fruit juice
1 oz. of cold cereal
2 oz. of cooked cereal, rice or pasta
8 oz. of milk or yogurt

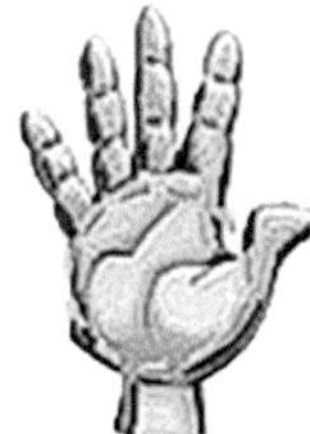

Palm = 3 oz. of meat

Choose lean poultry, fish, shellfish and beef. One palm size portion equals 3 oz. for an adult and 1½-2 oz. for a child under 5.

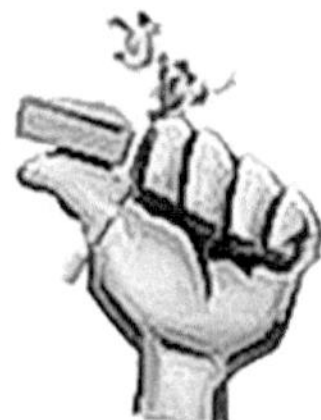

A thumb = 1 oz. of cheese

Consuming low fat cheese helps you meet the required servings from the milk, yogurt and cheese group. 1½ oz. of low fat cheese counts as 8 oz. of milk or yogurt.

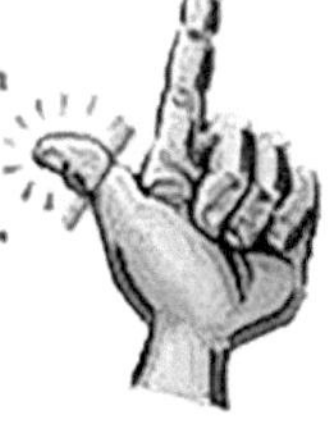

Thumb tip = 1 teaspoon

Keep high fat foods, such as peanut butter and mayonnaise, at a minimum. One teaspoon is equal to the end of your thumb, from the knuckle up. Three teaspoons equals 1 tablespoon.

Handful = 1-2 oz. of snack food

Snacking can add up. Remember, 1 handful equals 1 oz. of nuts and small candies. For chips and pretzels, 2 handfuls equal 1 oz.

1 tennis ball = ½ cup of fruit and vegetables

Healthy diets include a variety of colorful fruits and vegetables every day.

There are 2 questions that are likely crossing your mind right now:

1. **Who has the time?** Between commuting, work, and the kids, most people's hectic schedules leave barely enough time to sleep, let alone time to prepare 3 meals every day.
2. **How can anyone afford it?** Grocery bills are sky high the way it is. Adding all that organic, fresh food could send us to the poor house.

These arguments may seem real, now, but they're really false dilemmas.

There is one inescapable fact: if you aren't feeding your body the nutrition it needs to be healthy, your body is decomposing, and your health is declining.

- **Your body has a big job to do, and it depends on you for help.**

Your body works 24/7 to:

1. Energize and protect itself.
2. Replace millions of cells that, through a process called Apoptosis, are preprogrammed to die.
3. **Also, while your body is at it, it produces millions of other cells** damaged by the rigors of everyday life, **more cells** – due to normal wear and tear, brought on by work, **more cells** – due to excessive wear and tear, brought on by our penchant for strenuous exercise and recreation.

You get the picture; it's a monumental task and your body is challenged every day.

Question: Does your body have enough nutrition, consumed in your diet, to support the repair of damaged tissue and replacement of all the dead and dying cells – or not?

If there is sufficient nutrition – your body is regenerating.

. . . producing perfect cells and you are staying healthy.

If not – your body is decomposing

. . . the cells and tissue are produced and repaired imperfectly, and you are becoming less healthy. This decline in your health occurs in stages, over time, and it will culminate in an unhealthy state.

Caring for the needs of your body may be the most important task you have.

All those other things, that you have prioritized above treating your body kindly, won't matter once you have lost your health.

Neglecting your body catches up with you – sooner or later. The decline will start with nagging inconveniences such as: diminished energy, indigestion, food sensitivity, weight gain, irritability; escalating to some sort of "managed condition", using drug store preparations and/or one, or more, prescriptions: culminating in the miserable state of declining health.

When you lose your health – you'll lose everything. . . You can either: invest in your health now or pay dearly when you are not healthy later.

Note: As amazing as it may seem, most adults, teens, and children in this land of plenty are malnourished. Certainly, they're not starving, but they are lacking the basic nutrition their bodies require to function and flourish.

The Situation Isn't as Bleak as it Appears.

There are steps everyone can take to avoid the predictable outcome – not being healthy or failing health.

1. **First, Start Taking Care of Your Body's Nutritional Needs.** You know what to do … eat more healthfully … so, do the best you can.
   Note: There is one thing to remember … if you don't buy it, you can't eat it.
2. **Second, once you've done your best with your diet, fill the gaps in your diet with supplements**. Those gaps will likely be consuming enough raw, mineral rich vegetables and fruit. *Note:* the supplements to consider are Trace minerals, Enzymes and Phytonutrients from above ground vegetables, fruits, berries, grasses, and adding a general multivitamin.

These first two steps will address diet health issues going forward, . . . but there are residual nutritional deficiencies from past years.

Next, you need to undo the effects of the historic deficiencies of nutrition your body experienced. Choose supplements that address your specific health needs and will support the body's ability to restore that particular function.

Don't be surprised! The body will establish its priorities, and they may be different than your priorities. The good news is your body is beginning to restore itself, and your health, thanks to your decision to treat it kindly.

Be patient! The healing process is predictable, too. It takes about 1 month of treating your body respectfully for each year you have spent neglecting it.

- **No One is Going to Get Out of This Life – Alive.**

While the statistics are changing, most reputable sources proudly proclaim that life expectancy is longer now than at any other time in history.

It's true! You can expect to live longer than your grandparents.

But, at what cost? One of the fastest growing industries in the Industrialized World is managed health care.

That's right – managing people's declining health is big business! Dealing with the nagging complaints using non-prescription medications, managing the symptoms of declining health with doctors, specialists and prescriptions, housing and caring for the infirm, once the other treatments become ineffectual - IS BIG BUSINESS. **And it's growing**.

At every phase, along this predictable journey toward managed care, there are ethical companies producing aids to ease the suffering of the afflicted and caring, highly trained people, offering aid and comfort, working to stabilize the stages of declining health.

What's Missing?
The answer is the afflicted people think they do not need to be part of the effort. Too many people believe that "showing up" is enough; that technology and expertise will win the day.

Here's the travesty: the person who is beneficiary of the effort, often continues to practice the same dietary and lifestyle choices that delivered him or her to their predicament.

As of this writing, instances of lung cancer are decreasing in the general population.

The report rightly attributes the change to a person's choice to stop smoking. After all the suffering, effort and expense, lung cancer is succumbing to a lifestyle change – the decision to stop smoking.

Why? Because people started "getting it."

They started showing up - people stopped smoking.

That choice changed the predictable outcome: smoking increases instances of Lung Cancer.

People became part of the "*cure*" by making a different lifestyle choice.

- **Final thoughts** •

Your choices will put you on 1 of 2 predictable paths, too.

1. One is: Bad Nutrition Increases the Instances not Being Healthy.
2. The other is: Good Nutrition Equals Good Health.

It's your life – it's your choice. Choose wisely!

Lesson 4: Supplements

Question: Do you need to take supplements?

Answer: The difference between what you consume and what your body needs to stay healthy creates a gap that allows your health to leak away. The bigger the hole, the faster your health leaks away! Supplements fill those leaks. You decide!

Your Body Makes Beautiful Music

Health is the beautiful music that is produced when your body is functioning efficiently. It is the normal state of being when each section in your body's orchestra – digestion, circulation, metabolism, and others – is doing their part to keep you healthy, vibrant and youthful.

Health is Like a Symphony

A symphonic orchestra combines different instruments, strings, woodwinds, brass, and percussion to form an ensemble that has the potential to create beautiful music. Each musical arrangement blends the sound of the different instruments into a musical presentation that tantalizes the listener.

If, during a particular concert, one of the violinists happens to be absent, the other violinists can compensate for the missing person without affecting the concert—very much. And, even if a person from the trumpet section happens to be absent that night, the orchestra could adjust the presentation.

Health is the Normal Condition – It's Your Symphony of Health

Health is characterized by the body's ability to maintain efficient function. Your body depends on a consistent source of nutrients, called the balanced diet, to sustain that normal condition because the various tissues and components that make up your body wear out and can be damaged during the course of living.

Like the orchestra compensates for a missing musician, your body can compensate for missing nutrients, for a short period of time when the basic nutrients are missing – if it must.

What if an entire section of the orchestra doesn't show up? Can you imagine a symphony without violins, or trumpets? **That beautiful music would descend into noise.**

Unfortunately, once your body starts to compensate it begins to decay (the descent from health) . . . and, depending on the length of time and number of systems involved, you will experience different abnormal conditions.

Disease – and Failing Health – is an Abnormal Condition

Disease is characterized by a gradual degeneration of the body's ability to maintain normal function ... because your body lacks a reliable, sufficient source of nutrients to sustain and repair itself.

• Perform a Reality Check

When asked, almost everyone will say, "*I eat a pretty healthy diet.* "

People need to stop kidding themselves.

For most people, eating a balanced diet is an illusion. The combination of commuting to work, the demands at work or school, and family commitments make grabbing something on the way far easier than eating a healthy meal three times a day – or even once a day for that matter.

Whether your orchestra is missing a few musicians, or entire sections, your symphony of health – isn't beautiful music.

Natural supplements help fill the gap in your diet, so your body can produce the glorious symphony of health.

Lesson 5: Hand to Mouth Disease

- **Hand to Mouth Disease affects everyone sooner or later.**

You won't find this particular diagnosis anywhere, but you will find the symptoms described everywhere. They have diagnoses like being overweight or obese, constipation, digestive disorders, diabetes, hypertension, cardiovascular disease, osteoporosis, joint disease, cancer, and a whole host of complaints that are being managed – not cured.

The Causes of Hand to Mouth Disease

Eating a Balanced Diet Is a Myth. There are still people who believe they can rely on their diet for all the different nutrients to sustain a healthy body.

There was a time when that may have been true— but not now. There are too many things like: early harvest, GMO, agriculture chemicals, etc., that render this an improbability.

It's just – not likely.

Here's why.

For those of you who are trying to eat a balanced diet, keep it up! But know this about your Balanced Diet:

1. **The fresh foods you are eating have been grown on the same cropland over and over again**. These foods are likely lacking important trace minerals that have long since been depleted from the soil.
2. **Plus, the produce has been harvested early** so they can reach the supermarket and sold to you before it spoils.

These two situations are creating the gap between what your body needs and the nutrient availability in your diet. **And, when you cook this fresh food, you may be widening the gap even further** because sustained temperatures of 108° affect the viability of food enzymes in your fresh food.

For the rest of us who aren't eating the way we should - there is a direct correlation between your health and your diet. You either are or will be paying the price for neglecting your diet.

When you depend on packaged foods, you are also eating additives that:

- Maintain the "appealing look" of the food,
- Change the flavor, so it doesn't taste like it came from a package.
- Stop the contents from spoiling by interrupting any microbial action.

When this preservative action continues along the digestive tract, it is likely that the friendly microbes in your intestinal tract, that are responsible for the conversion of food to nutrients, are impacted as well.

There are other considerations for food additives, too.

Regulators have deemed these individual chemicals Generally Recognized as Safe (GRAS). However, we never eat these chemicals individually, they are part of a meal that usually consists of several different packaged foods containing different GRAS chemicals. And there is limited information concerning the impact of combining these GRAS chemicals, but the possibility exists that combining the different GRAS chemicals may be creating altogether different substances than those that have been studied.

For example, Refined grain (like white flour and white rice) peeled tubers (potatoes and other underground growing vegetables) and meat do not contain any fiber. Besides supporting timely elimination, fiber manages sugar, cholesterol, toxin accumulation and many other functions – without them, you're sure to have a slow or backed up sewer festering inside your body. Nutritionists universally suggest a minimum of 30 grams of dietary fiber, every day.

Breakfast cereal, a burger and fries for lunch and something quick for dinner doesn't even come close. There are some studies that suggest the lack of fiber in the typical diet may be contributing to digestive distress, cholesterol issues, sugar issues and certain cancers.

Hand to Mouth Disease is going to make you suffer before it kills you.

1. If that's your objective – suffer mightily before you die - then keep doing what you are doing.
2. **If dying sick is not your objective, then start changing the things you do.**

- **Choosing and Consuming food is your job!**

Whoever said: "*Breakfast is your most important meal" was right!*

You must eat breakfast to jump-start your body and that first 12 oz. glass of water is critical, and . . .

When You Wake Up Start Eating Breakfast.

How many of you have experienced a fast? You know, where you can't eat or drink anything for 8 to 12 hours. Can you remember how hungry and thirsty you were afterwards?

Your body experiences a fast every day – but, you don't think about it because you are sleeping. The thing is, your body is rebuilding, using energy from calories and the nutrients from your diet to repair your damaged and worn-out tissue while you are sleeping. After this daily fast, your body needs water and more energy.

Recipe for the Perfect Breakfast

1. Soak regular oatmeal in water overnight in a covered pan.
2. Add applesauce to thin and sweeten the oats.
3. Add 1 tsp. of flax seed oil.
4. Sprinkle 1 to 2 tsp. of cinnamon on the oats
5. Crumble 6 walnut halves on top of the oats.
6. If you must have a sweet flavor, use xylitol (sounds like a chemical – but it's not! It comes from a plant. It tastes like sugar, but it isn't - and it has been shown to help with dental cavities.

Start drinking water. The number 1 beneficial supplement is good 'ol water.

The formula for "enough water" is divide your body weight by 2 to determine the number of ounces of water you need to hydrate your body and flush out the waste. **Other liquids do not count!** If you drink caffeinated drinks, add 2 ounces of water for each ounce of caffeinated beverage.

Start eating real food. You should never be hungry. Eat more vegetables (all colors, raw, steamed and cooked to crunchy) that grow above the ground and less meat (about the size of a deck of cards would be perfect.) If you can't or won't, take a supplement.

Start snacking. Eat an apple or pear (every color there is) between meals. When you heard: "An apple a day keeps the Doctor away.", it was the truth.

Start losing weight.

Fad diets are a waste of time. Straightening your diet will go a long way in helping you lose weight. If you still need help, find a well- formulated weight management supplement to help with metabolism and cravings. Take your supplements religiously until the reflection in the mirror corresponds to the image you have in your mind.

Start taking multivitamins. Even the AMA recommends taking a multi-vitamin every day. Make sure your supplement(s) contains more than the RDI (recommended daily intake of nutrients) because that RDI level isn't enough to keep you healthy – it is just enough to keep you not sick.

And, while you're at it, make sure the pill(s) will dissolve in your body. Add a teaspoon of vinegar to an 8-ounce glass of tepid water (the temperature of formula you would feed a baby.), add the pill.

- If it dissolves in the glass, it will dissolve in your body.
- If not, you are wasting your money and you need to find a multi-vitamin that is better.

Editor's note: **I invest about $3.50 a day in supplements to help me stay healthy.** I'm 76 years old, seldom sick, take no prescriptions and keep up with our grandchildren. I avoid the typical land mines – smoking and drinking to excess and I enjoy life. I plan to die healthy. Can you say the same thing?

Make of this what you will. High quality dietary supplements aren't magic bullets . . . they aren't secret potions . . . they are supplements that are intended to fill the gap between what you are eating to make yourself not healthy and or sick and what you should be consuming to stay healthy.

Isn't that enough? NO? You want more?

Question: What if you find yourself dealing with something more than occasional inconveniences?

Answer: Hand to Mouth Disease is progressive. You may be suffering from the symptoms of the latter stages of the disorder – and they can be more frequent, moving toward severity, on to more profound condition.

In any case, the impact of the amount and/or type may be the culprit. Identifying and eliminating the culprit is important. The Exclusion Diet has helped hundreds of people identify, along with lifestyle mapping, the root cause of their persistent, nagging health challenge.

Even more people have used this approach to make radiant health their reality. Enjoy your experience of a renewed relationship with your body.

The Exclusion Diet

Do you Struggle with waning health, strange symptoms, or unexplainable illnesses?

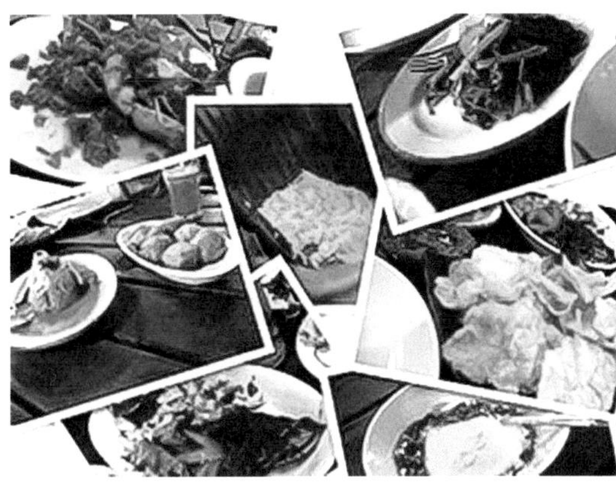

. . . If you're experiencing:

- **Bloating**
- **Indigestion**
- **Brain Fog**
- **Weight Gain**
- **Headache**
- **Strange Symptoms**
- **Diminished Vitality**

. . . food sensitivities might be the culprit.

They're not really food allergies – nor are they as profound as anaphylaxis, but food sensitivities are very disagreeable!

The process of elimination, in the Exclusion Diet, helps people identify the subtle – sometimes gradual – reactions to the foods – common to their diet – that are, more than likely, causing their strange symptoms.

The Exclusion Diet is like pushing the "reset" button for food sensitivities and strange symptoms.

During a short 2 weeks, the exclusion diet helps your body clear out any sensitivities and the antibodies that the body has produced over time. Most people feel dramatically better, and they may even lose some weight!

Afterwards, you add each food you have excluded – one by one – to test whether the body's response is good or bad – and the mystery will be solved.

Here's the food that you should eliminate to start with:

Gluten (wheat, rye, and barley)	Eggs	Dairy, milk, cheese, yog
Soy	Corn	Peanuts
Sugar (table, tropical fruit, fruit juice)	Vinegar	Alcohol
All artificial preservatives, additives, dyes, sweeteners, etc.		

IMPORTANT: Many people have food sensitivities to more than one food. So, unless you eliminate all these foods, you may not notice a difference in how you feel, or you won't necessarily see improvement.

The Only Rule for the Exclusion Diet is: Failing to Plan is - Planning to Fail.

. . . SO, make a grocery list AND BUY the foods you CAN eat such as:

1. Organic meat protein sources (fish, chicken, bison, beef)
2. Healthy fats like avocado butter, coconut oil or coconut butter, olive oil, nut oils and grape seed oil.
3. Make sure to get a variety of fresh green and colorful vegetables that grow above the ground, and apples and pears – and vow to try something new every day!
4. Milk alternatives, like coconut milk and almond milk
5. Lemon or Lime Juice (to replace vinegar)
6. Be sure to stock up on snack foods like apples, pears, raw nuts, seeds, and nut butters.
7. Then, plan meals, eat a wide variety of whole foods and do not restrict your calorie intake.
   NOTE: If you don't experience an improvement with your strange symptoms associated with food sensitivities during the 2 weeks, you either don't have any food sensitivities or you may need further testing, such as acid testing or a comprehensive analysis for parasites.

After the 2 weeks, you can start to reintroduce the foods that you have excluded.

It is VERY important to do so one by one, with only one new food introduced every 2-3 days. That way you can monitor your body for return of symptoms, such as brain fog, water retention, or bloating. If you notice symptoms with a certain food, take that one back out and try something else.

The Exclusion Diet will provide you with a sense of what foods agree with you – and which ones make you feel terrible. You decide what you are willing to tolerate then continue avoiding the foods that make you feel the worst.

Changing habits, especially involving food, can be difficult - I promise you the health reward will be well worth it. And soon you'll be feeling so much better that you will not even miss the foods you've given up!

Exclusion Diet – Issues & FAQ's

Q: What if you're still hungry?

A: If you find yourself hungry during the elimination diet, first ask yourself "Am I really hungry?"

There are other reasons people eat like: boredom, emotions, and fatigue.

If you are not experiencing any of these and you're still hungry, you are probably not eating enough fat. Increase your intake of healthy fats like avocado on top of burgers, or try adding walnut, sesame, or coconut oil on top of roasted veggies and vegetable salads. Plus, you can snack on nuts, nut butter or coconut butter dips for meat and vegetables.

The first few days will be the hardest as your body goes through withdrawal from sugar and your cravings will be more intense or your strange symptoms might intensify.

Symptoms you may experience in the first week or so can include changes in sleep patterns, lightheadedness, headaches, joint or muscle stiffness and changes in gastrointestinal function. Such symptoms rarely last for more than a few days. It's called A Healing Crisis. You can read about it next!

You may find yourself walking around looking for something to eat and nothing sounds good.

This is usually because we have trained ourselves to snack on processed sugary foods, especially when we are bored or tired! You can drink a vegan safe, non-dairy, vitamin and mineral enriched shake to help. And be sure to start your day with a healthy vegan-safe breakfast shake mixed with almond or coconut milk, too.

Q. What do you do – after you finish the 2-week Exclusion Diet? A. The goal of the Exclusion Diet is to reconnect you to how food makes you feel.

There is no typical or normal response, and each person may differ in how they feel. The key is that you reestablish your connection with food and begin to understand how food affects the way you feel.

Exclusion Diet – Grey Area Foods

The purpose of the exclusion diet is to identify foods that may be affecting your health. This means avoiding all grains, legumes, and dairy products as well as refined sugar, processed food chemicals and modern vegetable oils. Many advocates of the exclusion diet suggest eliminating all gray area foods, too.

Note: Gray area foods are especially important factors if you are suffering from immune system issues or a history of poor gut health. You may choose to avoid these foods in your implementation of the exclusion diet.

The main grey area culprits are:

Nuts and Seeds: Nuts and seeds contain small amounts of gut irritants (saponins) and anti-nutrients (phytates, which inhibit the absorption of vitamins and minerals). Note: The phytate content can be minimized by soaking nuts and seeds overnight - then drying them in the oven at low temperature or in a food dehydrator - before consuming them. Most nuts and seeds also contain more omega-6 fatty acids than omega-3 fatty acids (ratios ranging from 1:3 to 1:10), which isn't helpful as we strive for a 1:1 ratio of omega-3 to omega-6 fatty acids in our diets.

Dairy products from Cows and Goats: Dairy products are blacklisted for two reasons: (1) They can irritate the gut in some people and (2) they cause a spike in your insulin disproportional to the amount of sugar in milk (even cheese, which is mostly protein and fat, spikes your insulin).

Important: These issues may be reduced – but not eliminated - in goat dairy and in dairy from pasture-fed cows. Plus, many people can tolerate these. The bonus of dairy from pasture-fed cows is that it contains Conjugated Linoleic Acid and more omega-3 fatty acids – unfortunately, it's hard to find.

Nightshades (Peppers, Eggplants, Tomatoes and Potatoes): Vegetables in this family contain small amounts of poisonous glycoalkaloids (tomatine, solanine and chaconine).
Note: You may or may not be sensitive to these chemicals, depending on your lineage. A way to minimize your exposure is to eat the ripest version of the vegetable (ripe tomatoes, red bell peppers, etc. Note: potatoes seem to be especially problematic, so many exclusion dieters avoid potatoes even if they include the other nightshades in their diet. If you do want to eat potatoes, peeling them gets rid of most of the glycoalkaloids.

Eggs: Eggs can be problematic for some people. A chemical called lysozyme in the egg white can form globs of molecules in the gut and sneak things across the gut lining that shouldn't be able to get into your blood stream.
Note: Isn't it strange to realize that egg yolks are the healthy part of the egg - especially when you eat omega-3 or free-range eggs?

Caffeine: Coffee and other caffeinated beverages increase your cortisol (stress hormone) levels. Most of us are trying to reduce stress, not increase it, so large amounts of caffeine are problematic.
Note: You could try green tea. Important: If you cannot eliminate coffee: It helps to drink coffee black (the fat in cream increases how quickly the caffeine gets into your blood stream) or with coconut creamer or almond milk.

Alcohol: The issue with alcohol is dose. Alcohol is a toxin, and it increases your blood triglycerides and your risk of cardiovascular disease. If you are having issues with sleep quality, cut alcoholic beverages out completely.
Note: If you can't eliminate alcohol, limit yourself to one or two drinks at a time, no more than a couple of times per week – or less. Important: Most beer contains gluten - Spirits generally don't. Many wines contain preservatives – refer to label.

Consider all these grey area foods as possible culprits for continued health issues as you experiment with the exclusion diet.

Conclusion

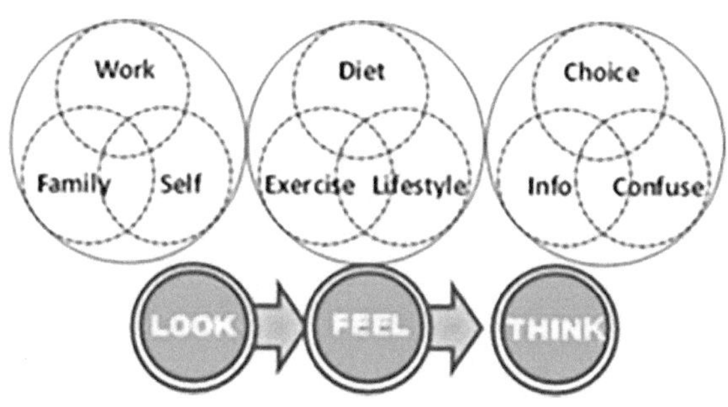

21st Living is like driving a 3-wheel chariot down an unfamiliar road toward a "to be announced" destination.

Your job is to keep the wheels balanced and the chariot on the road.

Your choices are too much, too little, and just right. Choosing "just right" keeps you out of the ditch and on time.

Sounds simple – but it's not easy. Let's make this easier.

Humans are diurnal.

Humans are active during the day (after sunup) and need sleep at night (after sundown).

There are unlimited choices for food that Humans can consume. The earth offers abundant water, plants, fish, birds, and small and large beasts that are edible. Plants offer leaves, nuts, fruit, berries, bulbs, and seeds that are edible. Beasts produce meat that is edible.

Your ancestors survived because they learned what to do:

- They ate the produce of plants that they were collecting and storing and the meat from animals they were about to trap or occasional big beast hunt.
- They walked to collect, trap, and hunt their food and they walked to nearby streams to collect water – transporting manageable loads by hand back to their compound.
- They established small cohorts of other competent and worthy humans for protection and companionship.

- They ate and collaborated by the light of a fire at night - retiring to their shelter to sleep until sunrise. Then they awoke and repeated the process.
- They survived life or death confrontations with individuals and marauding raiders.
- They selected mates to produce offspring whom they protected, nurtured, and trained to be new members of human society.
- Their offspring, in turn, repeated the process throughout the generations of humans - that produced you.

Genetics rule the day.

Frank Booth, a biologist and geneticist, who teaches in the College of Veterinary Medicine at the University of Missouri at Columbia reports: *"Technology has changed, but our genes have not. Ten thousand years ago, we had to go out and search for food and get food. Now, we have those same genes working – while you're waiting in the drive-through lane."*

So, here you are. . . the epitome of your ancestral line - living the 21st Century Lifestyle with Cave Man genetics.

Question: So, what do you do?

Answer: You compensate.

1. Change the things you can change (or find a work-around) and ignore the rest.
2. There are some things that won't change like instincts, nutrition, sleep, private time, meaningful, lasting companionship, emotions, and the drive to reproduce – manage them.

These mismatches between what your version 1 body needs and what you are presently delivering are the root cause of many of the chronic conditions afflicting your well-being.

Lifestyle mapping helps you identify those mismatches between your choices and the needs of your body. Once the mismatches are identified, resolved – and with enough time, your body is fully capable of restoring its genetically preferred state – healthy.

Question: What else?

Hint: There are 24 hours each day. The first Ven is work, family and self. It's a simple equation: 24 hours divided by 3 (the aspects of the first Ven) equals 8.

Then, allot your time like this: 8 for work, 8 for family and friends, 8 for yourself. That is a perfect scenario. The hub of the wheel is in perfect harmony.

Do you see any balance issues in your Life Vens? I'll bet you do.

Your map will help you identify all the mismatches between your Version 1 body's needs and the 21st century lifestyle. Fix it – or develop a work-around to mitigate the conflict(s).

- **Simple enough.**

I'm positive you'll find it informative and a wonderful tool for taking control of your well-being. Enjoy the exercise of mapping your lifestyle. It will open your eyes - and your choices when negotiating the pathways for protecting and/or restoring your health.

Instructions and Journals for Lifestyle Mapping

Lifestyle mapping is a diary recording everything you do and feel during the day.

The purpose is simple: provide a statistically relevant study to determine the things that are affecting your body's ability to promote and maintain your health and well-being. **Ideally, it should be a 14-day study.** *IMPORTANT:* Do not change anything you would normally do.

Carefully print or copy one double-sided map, from the included mapping pages.

Copy (double-sided if possible) enough diary pages so you can add the information each day.

Note: if appropriate, attach a blank piece(s) of dated blank paper, if you need to record additional information.

Record everything you do and feel during the 14 days of study.

Once the study is complete, the lifestyle map will show a correlation between how you feel in the present to what you did – often habitually - in the past 24 hours that impact the *"sweet spot for balance"* - in either or both Vens - that are impacting your health and well-being.

At this point, it's up to you. In most cases the source of the issues you're experiencing will be glaring.

You need to adjust the imbalance(s). Develop a lifestyle strategy that will support living in harmony with the needs of your body (as discussed earlier) using the lifestyle journal.

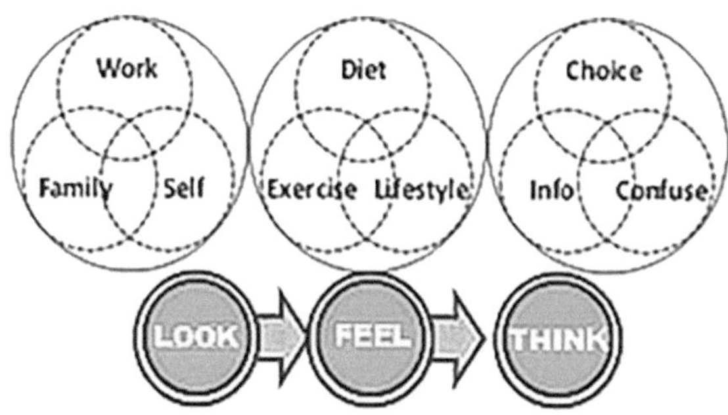

Note: If you're confused or have questions, it's likely your Physician won't have any answers. You'll need to contact a competent Holistic Health Practitioner or Natural Health Consultant to help you interpret the findings of your study.

Question: Will you heed your body's cry for help and become a partner in the process - or not?

Hold this thought before you answer: Why not treat your body with the love, care, and respect that it deserves?

After all, you will only get one body, so it needs to last for your whole lifetime.

Answer: Choose wisely. **It's Your Life – it's Your Choice. Enjoy the Experience.**

Following are pages for your daily journal.

Note: Most people prefer to copy 2 weeks' worth of pages so, in the future, you can repeat the process if need be.

Day				
Awake	**Breakfast**	**Lunch**	**Diner**	**Bed**
Time	**Time**	**Time**	**Time**	**Time**
How do you feel?				
Oz. of H_2O consumed during the day?				
Meals and Snacks Everything!				
Describe your day.				

Day				
Awake	**Breakfast**	**Lunch**	**Diner**	**Bed**
Time	**Time**	**Time**	**Time**	**Time**
How do you feel?				
Oz. of H_2O consumed during the day?				
Meals and Snacks Everything!				
Describe your day.				

Day				
Awake	**Breakfast**	**Lunch**	**Diner**	**Bed**
Time	**Time**	**Time**	**Time**	**Time**
How do you feel?				
Oz. of H_2O consumed during the day?				
Meals and Snacks Everything!				
Describe your day.				

Day				
Awake	**Breakfast**	**Lunch**	**Diner**	**Bed**
Time	**Time**	**Time**	**Time**	**Time**
How do you feel?				
Oz. of H_2O consumed during the day?				
Meals and Snacks Everything!				
Describe your day.				

Day				
Awake	**Breakfast**	**Lunch**	**Diner**	**Bed**
Time	**Time**	**Time**	**Time**	**Time**
How do you feel?				
Oz. of H_2O consumed during the day?				
Meals and Snacks Everything!				
Describe your day.				

Day				
Awake	**Breakfast**	**Lunch**	**Diner**	**Bed**
Time	**Time**	**Time**	**Time**	**Time**
How do you feel?				
Oz. of H_2O consumed during the day?				
Meals and Snacks Everything!				
Describe your day.				

Day				
Awake	**Breakfast**	**Lunch**	**Diner**	**Bed**
Time	**Time**	**Time**	**Time**	**Time**
How do you feel?				
Oz. of H_2O consumed during the day?				
Meals and Snacks Everything!				
Describe your day.				

Day				
Awake	**Breakfast**	**Lunch**	**Diner**	**Bed**
Time	**Time**	**Time**	**Time**	**Time**
How do you feel?				
Oz. of H_2O consumed during the day?				
Meals and Snacks Everything!				
Describe your day.				

Day				
Awake	**Breakfast**	**Lunch**	**Diner**	**Bed**
Time	**Time**	**Time**	**Time**	**Time**
How do you feel?				
Oz. of H_2O consumed during the day?				
Meals and Snacks Everything!				
Describe your day.				

Day				
Awake	**Breakfast**	**Lunch**	**Diner**	**Bed**
Time	**Time**	**Time**	**Time**	**Time**
How do you feel?				
Oz. of H_2O consumed during the day?				
Meals and Snacks Everything!				
Describe your day.				

Printed by Libri Plureos GmbH in Hamburg,
Germany